## Ashley Fitzgerald

# SOMATIC THERAPY
# FOR
# SEX IMPROVEMENT

**Transform Your Sex Life Through Mind-Body Practices**

© 2024 by Ashley Fitzgerald
© 2024 by UNITEXTO


**Published by UNITEXTO**

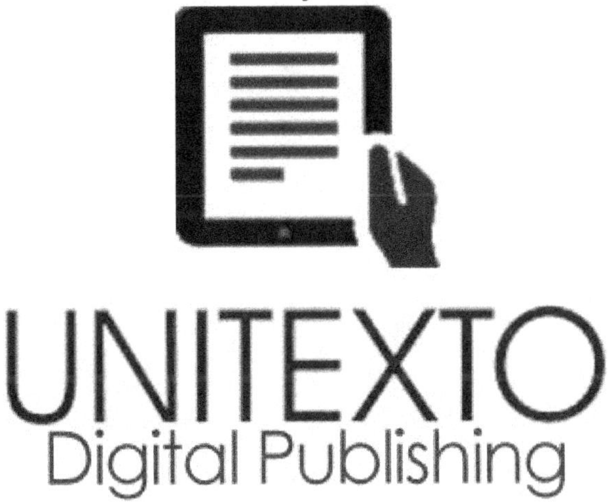

# TABLE OF CONTENTS

- Exploring the connection between sensation, emotion, and pleasure
- Practices for enhancing sensitivity and receptivity to touch

## Chapter 5: Breathwork and Sexual Energy
- Understanding the role of breath in sexual experiences and intimacy
- Exploring techniques for harnessing and channeling sexual energy through breathwork
- Breathwork exercises for relaxation, arousal, and intimacy enhancement

## Chapter 6: Movement and Expression in Sexual Pleasure
- The connection between movement, expression, and sexual pleasure
- Exploring somatic practices such as dance, yoga, and tai chi for enhancing sexual experiences
- Techniques for cultivating body confidence and freedom of expression in the bedroom

## Chapter 7: Healing Trauma and Resolving Blockages
- Addressing the impact of past traumas and negative experiences on sexual health
- Techniques for somatic healing and releasing emotional and physical blockages
- Strategies for creating a safe and supportive environment for sexual healing

## Chapter 8: Partner Communication and Connection
- The importance of open and honest communication in sexual relationships
- Techniques for enhancing intimacy, trust, and connection with a partner
- Exercises for deepening emotional and physical intimacy through somatic practices

## Chapter 9: Sensory Exploration and Erotic Play
- Exploring the role of sensory stimulation in sexual pleasure
- Techniques for incorporating sensory exploration and erotic play into sexual experiences
- Mindful approaches to exploring fantasies, desires, and boundaries with a partner

## Chapter 10: Cultivating Presence and Mindfulness in Sexual Encounters
- The practice of mindfulness in the context of sexual intimacy
- Techniques for cultivating presence, awareness, and mindfulness during sexual encounters
- Mindful approaches to arousal, pleasure, and orgasm

## Chapter 11: Integrating Somatic Therapy into Daily Life
- Strategies for integrating somatic therapy practices into everyday routines
- Techniques for maintaining sexual health and vitality outside of the bedroom
- Creating a holistic approach to sexual well-being through somatic awareness

## Chapter 12: Embracing Sexual Liberation and Empowerment
- Celebrating sexual diversity, pleasure, and liberation
- Embracing individuality and self-expression in sexual experiences
- Strategies for ongoing growth, exploration, and empowerment in sexuality

## Chapter 13: Somatic Practices for Couples
-Utilizing somatic techniques to enhance sexual experiences as a couple

-Building trust, communication, and intimacy through shared somatic practices

**Chapter 14. Academic research:**
-Academic Open Access Journals
-Searching key words

# Why This Book?

In a world filled with endless information and advice on sexuality, relationships, and personal growth, you might be wondering, "Why this book?" What sets SOMATIC THERAPY FOR SEX IMPROVEMENT apart from the myriad of options available to you?

This book is not just another self-help manual or a guide to sexual techniques. It's a journey—a journey of self-discovery, empowerment, and transformation. It's an invitation to explore the depths of your desires, confront your fears, and embrace your authenticity in all its complexity.

So why this book? Because it dares to challenge the status quo, to question societal norms and expectations, and to celebrate the beauty and diversity of human sexuality. It's a book that acknowledges that there is no one-size-fits-all approach to sex and relationships, and that each individual's journey is unique and valid.

Through a blend of practical advice, personal anecdotes, and thought-provoking reflections, SOMATIC THERAPY FOR SEX IMPROVEMENT guides you on a path of exploration and discovery, helping you navigate the complexities of modern sexuality with confidence and grace. Whether you're seeking to enhance your intimate relationships, overcome sexual challenges, or simply deepen your understanding of yourself, this book offers valuable insights and tools to support you every step of the way.

Some reasons to buy and read this book:

1. **Embrace Authenticity:**

This book encourages readers to embrace their authentic selves, challenging societal norms and expectations surrounding sexuality. By delving into the complexities of desire, identity, and pleasure, readers can gain a deeper understanding of themselves and their unique sexual journeys.

2. **Navigate Modern Relationships:**
In today's ever-evolving world, navigating relationships can be challenging. This book offers practical advice and insights to help readers navigate the complexities of modern relationships with confidence and grace. Whether you're single, in a partnership, or exploring alternative relationship structures, this book provides valuable guidance for fostering healthy, fulfilling connections.

3. **Expand Your Sexual Horizons:**
Whether you're looking to enhance intimacy with a partner or explore new realms of pleasure on your own, this book offers a wealth of information and inspiration. From communication techniques to sensual exploration exercises, readers will discover practical tools to expand their sexual horizons and cultivate deeper connections with themselves and others.

4. **Overcome Sexual Challenges:**
Many individuals face obstacles on their sexual journey, from performance anxiety to communication barriers. This book provides compassionate support and practical strategies for overcoming common sexual challenges, empowering readers to reclaim agency over their bodies and experiences.

5. **Foster Self-Discovery and Growth:**

Beyond the realm of sexuality, this book encourages readers to embark on a journey of self-discovery and personal growth. Through reflective exercises, journal prompts, and thought-provoking insights, readers can explore their desires, fears, and aspirations, ultimately leading to greater self-awareness and fulfillment.

6. **Celebrate Diversity and Inclusivity:**
   This book celebrates the diversity of human sexuality and honors the multitude of identities and experiences within the LGBTQ+ community and beyond. By centering diverse voices and perspectives, this book fosters a culture of inclusivity and acceptance, inviting readers of all backgrounds to participate in the conversation.

7. **Cultivate Empowerment:**
   Ultimately, this book is a celebration of sexual empowerment and liberation. By reclaiming agency over their bodies and experiences, readers can cultivate a sense of empowerment that transcends societal expectations and limitations. Through self-acceptance, self-expression, and self-love, readers can embark on a journey of empowerment that extends far beyond the pages of this book.

Whether you're seeking guidance on navigating relationships, exploring your sexuality, or simply embarking on a journey of self-discovery, SOMATIC THERAPY FOR SEX IMPROVEMENT offers invaluable insights and inspiration to support you on your path..

So, if you're ready to embark on a journey of self-discovery and sexual empowerment, if you're ready to challenge the norms and expectations that society has placed upon you, then this book is for you. Because ultimately, the question is not "Why this book?" but rather, "Why not?"

**Ashley Fitzgerald**

## About the Author:

Ashley Fitzgerald: An Embodiment of Healing and Personal Triumph
From a tender age, I, Ashley Fitzgerald, was acutely attuned to the nuances of health and personal well-being. These early inklings of self-awareness were not just passing contemplations but the seeds of a lifelong journey towards self-improvement and healing.

As the chapters of life unfolded, I embraced my calling with fervor, transforming my youthful concerns into a robust career that spans two decades. Today, I stand before you not merely as a practitioner but as a seasoned professional healer whose hands and heart have been instrumental in guiding countless individuals towards weight loss triumphs, enriched sexual health, and the surmounting of life's multifaceted challenges to reach the pinnacle of their health aspirations.

My professional and academic journey is a tapestry of diverse yet interconnected disciplines. With an insatiable thirst for knowledge, I delved deep into the realms of yoga and meditation, not just as practices but as academic pursuits, seeking to understand their profound effects on the human psyche and physiology.

This spiritual and intellectual quest further led me to the healing energies of Reiki, the organic wisdom in health foods, and the transformative potential of neuroscience and positive psychology.

My foray into the science of health and exercise is not merely academic; it is a reflection of my intrinsic philosophy that the body and mind are inextricable partners in the dance of life.

My dedication to personal growth extends beyond my professional endeavors—it is a way of life. Each morning, as the world stirs awake, I find sanctuary in my daily rituals. My practice of yoga is more than a physical regimen; it is a journey towards achieving a state of zen-like tranquility, a testament to my belief in the power of simplicity and inner peace. Meditation accompanies yoga as my mental compass, guiding me through life's tumultuous waves with a steadfast calm.

What fuels my unyielding passion is an unwavering drive—an innate desire to not only absorb the myriad teachings that life has to offer but also to disseminate them. I am imbued with a relentless drive to unearth and share life strategies that spark a transformative flame within souls, urging them to reach for health, well-being, and the fruition of their deepest dreams.

It was this very desire that led me to the world of writing, to become a scribe of my experiences and insights. My pen is driven by a profound commitment to be a beacon of positivity, influencing the lives of others through words that resonate with truth and vitality.

As you turn the pages of my books, what you will find is a reflection of my heart's work. I invite you into my world, not just as a reader, but as a fellow traveler on this grand adventure of life. Thank you for embarking on this journey with me, and it is my sincerest hope that you will find as much joy in reading my writings as I found in penning them down. May the words you peruse inspire you to cultivate the health and happiness you so richly deserve.

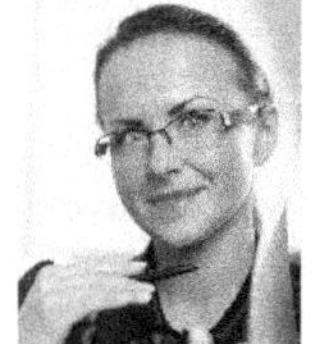

**Ashley Fitzgerald**

## Chapter 1: Introduction to Somatic Therapy for Sexual Enhancement

- Defining somatic therapy and its application in the realm of sexual health
- Overview of the mind-body connection in sexual experiences
- Introducing the concept of somatic awareness and its role in sexual fulfillment

Sexuality is a fundamental aspect of human experience, encompassing a wide range of emotions, sensations, and desires. Yet, for many individuals, achieving sexual fulfillment can be elusive, hindered by factors such as stress, trauma, and societal expectations. In recent years, somatic therapy has emerged as a promising approach to addressing sexual concerns and enhancing intimacy. This chapter serves as an introduction to somatic therapy for sexual enhancement, exploring its theoretical underpinnings, practical applications, and potential benefits.

### Defining Somatic Therapy:

Somatic therapy, also known as somatic experiencing or somatic psychology, is a holistic approach to healing that focuses on the interconnectedness of mind, body, and spirit. Rooted in the belief that the body holds wisdom and memory, somatic therapy aims to release physical tension, trauma, and emotional blockages stored within the body. Through a combination of mindfulness practices, body awareness techniques, and gentle movement exercises, somatic therapy seeks to restore balance and vitality to the individual.

Dr. Peter Levine, a pioneering figure in somatic therapy, describes it as follows: "Somatic experiencing is a body-oriented approach to the healing of trauma and other stress disorders. It is based on the observation that wild animals, though threatened routinely, are rarely traumatized." This observation underscores the innate capacity of the body to regulate and heal itself when provided with the necessary support and resources.

**The Mind-Body Connection in Sexual Experiences:**

At the heart of somatic therapy lies the recognition of the profound connection between the mind and body in shaping our experiences, including those of a sexual nature. Research in the fields of psychology and neuroscience has provided ample evidence of the intricate interplay between physical sensations, emotional states, and cognitive processes during sexual arousal and intimacy.

Dr. Esther Perel, a renowned psychotherapist and author, emphasizes this connection, stating: "Our bodies are not just transporters of brains, they are integral parts of our mind." In the context of sexuality, this means that our physical experiences, such as touch, movement, and breath, are inextricably linked to our emotional and psychological responses.

**Introducing Somatic Awareness:**

Somatic awareness refers to the ability to tune into and consciously experience the sensations, emotions, and energies present within the body. It involves cultivating a deep sense of self-awareness and attunement to one's internal landscape, including subtle cues and signals that may arise during sexual encounters.

Dr. Raja Selvam, a leading expert in somatic psychology, defines somatic awareness as "the capacity to attend to, feel, and track the sensations, movements, and energetic shifts that arise in the body moment by moment." This capacity forms the foundation of somatic therapy, enabling individuals to explore and transform their relationship with their bodies and themselves.

**Case Studies:**

To illustrate the potential of somatic therapy in enhancing sexual fulfillment, let us consider the following case studies:

Case Study 1:
Sarah, a 35-year-old woman, has been struggling with low libido and difficulty experiencing pleasure during sexual activity. Through somatic therapy sessions focused on breathwork and body awareness, Sarah learns to connect with her sensations and desires more fully. Over time, she begins to experience increased arousal and enjoyment in her intimate encounters, leading to greater satisfaction and intimacy in her relationship.

Case Study 2:
John, a 45-year-old man, has been grappling with performance anxiety and erectile dysfunction. Through somatic therapy sessions incorporating gentle movement exercises and mindfulness practices, John learns to release tension and relax into his body. As a result, he experiences greater ease and confidence in his sexual interactions, leading to improved erectile function and intimacy with his partner.

**Academic Papers and Books:**

For those interested in delving deeper into the theory and practice of somatic therapy for sexual enhancement, the following academic papers and books are recommended:

1. "In an Unspoken Voice: How the Body Releases Trauma and Restores Goodness" by Peter A. Levine
2. "The Body Keeps the Score: Brain, Mind, and Body in the Healing of Trauma" by Bessel van der Kolk
3. "The Tao of Sexology: The Book of Infinite Wisdom" by Dr. Stephen T. Chang
4. "Somatic Psychotherapy Toolbox: 125 Worksheets and Exercises to Treat Trauma & Stress" by Manuela Mischke-Reeds
5. "The Multi-Orgasmic Couple: Sexual Secrets Every Couple Should Know" by Mantak Chia and Douglas Abrams

**Exercises to Perform:**

To cultivate somatic awareness and enhance sexual fulfillment, consider incorporating the following exercises into your daily routine:

1. Body Scan Meditation:
   Take a few minutes each day to scan your body from head to toe, noticing any areas of tension or discomfort. Breathe deeply into these areas, allowing them to soften and release.
2. Sensory Exploration:
   Experiment with different textures, temperatures, and sensations on your skin, such as silk, velvet, or feathers. Notice how your body responds to each stimulus.
3. Breathwork Practice:
   Practice deep, slow breathing during moments of relaxation and intimacy. Focus on extending your exhale to promote relaxation and arousal.
4. Movement Meditation:
   Engage in gentle movement practices such as yoga, tai chi, or qigong to connect with your body and cultivate a sense of flow and vitality.

5.  Erotic Mapping:
    Take time to explore your own body and erogenous zones, noting what feels pleasurable and arousing. Share this information with your partner to enhance mutual understanding and intimacy.

## Conclusion:

In conclusion, somatic therapy offers a powerful framework for enhancing sexual fulfillment by fostering awareness, connection, and healing within the body. By embracing the mind-body connection and cultivating somatic awareness, individuals can unlock new levels of pleasure, intimacy, and satisfaction in their sexual experiences. Through the integration of theory, practice, and personal exploration, somatic therapy holds the potential to revolutionize our understanding and approach to sexuality.

**Chapter 2: Understanding Sexual Anatomy and Physiology**
- Exploring the intricacies of sexual anatomy in both men and women
- Understanding the physiological responses involved in sexual arousal and satisfaction
- Discussing common misconceptions and myths surrounding sexual anatomy and function

Sexual anatomy and physiology play a crucial role in shaping our experiences of pleasure, intimacy, and satisfaction. Understanding the intricacies of the human body in relation to sexual function is essential for cultivating healthy and fulfilling relationships. In this chapter, we delve into the fascinating world of sexual anatomy and physiology, exploring the physiological responses involved in sexual arousal and satisfaction, debunking common misconceptions, and highlighting the importance of sexual health education.

**Exploring Sexual Anatomy:**

Sexual anatomy encompasses a diverse array of structures and organs that contribute to the experience of pleasure and arousal in both men and women. In men, key anatomical features include the penis, testes, and prostate gland, while women possess the clitoris, vulva, vagina, and uterus. Each of these structures plays a unique role in the sexual response cycle, from arousal to orgasm and beyond.

Dr. Beverly Whipple, a pioneering researcher in the field of sexual physiology, emphasizes the importance of understanding sexual anatomy: "Knowledge of one's own body and sexual response is fundamental to sexual health and well-being. By exploring and understanding our anatomy, we can better appreciate the intricacies of sexual pleasure and function."

## Understanding Physiological Responses:

Sexual arousal and satisfaction are complex processes that involve a cascade of physiological responses throughout the body. In both men and women, sexual arousal is characterized by increased blood flow to the genital region, resulting in engorgement of erectile tissue and heightened sensitivity to touch and stimulation.

Dr. William H. Masters and Virginia E. Johnson, renowned sex researchers, describe the sexual response cycle as consisting of four stages: excitement, plateau, orgasm, and resolution. Each stage is accompanied by specific physiological changes, such as increased heart rate, muscle tension, and release of neurotransmitters such as dopamine and oxytocin.

## Discussing Misconceptions and Myths:

Despite advances in sexual health education, many misconceptions and myths persist regarding sexual anatomy and function. Common myths include the belief that vaginal orgasms are superior to clitoral orgasms, or that men must always achieve erection to experience sexual pleasure. These misconceptions can contribute to feelings of inadequacy, shame, and performance anxiety in individuals.

Dr. Emily Nagoski, author of "Come as You Are: The Surprising New Science that Will Transform Your Sex Life," challenges these myths, stating: "There is no one 'right' or 'normal' way to experience sexual pleasure. Each person's sexual response is unique and valid, and there is no hierarchy of orgasms or sexual experiences."

## Case Studies:

To illustrate the importance of understanding sexual anatomy and physiology, let us consider the following case studies:

Case Study 1:
Mark, a 30-year-old man, has been struggling with erectile dysfunction and performance anxiety. Through education about sexual anatomy and the physiological processes involved in arousal, Mark gains a deeper understanding of his body and sexual response. With this knowledge, he feels more confident and empowered to explore intimacy with his partner, leading to improved sexual satisfaction and communication.

Case Study 2:
Sarah, a 25-year-old woman, has been experiencing pain during intercourse and difficulty achieving orgasm. After learning about the anatomy of the clitoris and the role of arousal in reducing discomfort, Sarah begins to prioritize her own pleasure and communicate her needs to her partner. As a result, she experiences greater satisfaction and enjoyment in her sexual experiences.

**Academic Papers and Books:**

For those interested in further exploring sexual anatomy and physiology, the following academic papers and books are recommended:

1. "Human Sexual Response" by William H. Masters and Virginia E. Johnson
2. "The Clitoral Truth: The Secret World at Your Fingertips" by Rebecca Chalker
3. "Atlas of Human Sexual Anatomy" by C. David Tollison
4. "Sexual Anatomy and Physiology for Nurses" by Scott Jacoby

5. "The Science of Orgasm" by Barry R. Komisaruk, Beverly Whipple, and Carlos Beyer-Flores

**Exercises to Perform:**

To deepen your understanding of sexual anatomy and physiology, consider incorporating the following exercises into your routine:

1. Self-Exploration:
   Take time to explore your own body and become familiar with your own anatomy, including erogenous zones and areas of sensitivity.
2. Communication Practice:
   Practice discussing sexual anatomy and function with a partner or trusted friend, sharing questions, concerns, and insights openly and honestly.
3. Sensate Focus:
   Engage in sensate focus exercises with a partner, focusing on touch, sensation, and pleasure without the goal of orgasm or intercourse.
4. Anatomy Study:
   Use anatomical diagrams or educational resources to study sexual anatomy in detail, identifying key structures and their functions.
5. Mindful Touch:
   Practice mindful touch during solo or partnered sexual experiences, paying attention to sensations and responses in your body without judgment or expectation.

**Conclusion:**

In conclusion, understanding sexual anatomy and physiology is essential for cultivating healthy, fulfilling sexual relationships.

By exploring the intricacies of the human body and debunking common misconceptions, individuals can gain a deeper appreciation for their own sexual experiences and enhance intimacy with their partners. Through education, communication, and self-exploration, we can empower ourselves to embrace our sexuality fully and create more satisfying and fulfilling sexual connections.

## Chapter 3: The Role of Somatic Therapy in Addressing Sexual Dysfunction

- Identifying common sexual dysfunctions such as erectile dysfunction, premature ejaculation, and anorgasmia
- Exploring how somatic therapy techniques can help individuals overcome these challenges
- Case studies and examples of somatic therapy interventions for sexual dysfunction

Sexual dysfunction is a prevalent issue that can significantly impact an individual's quality of life and intimate relationships. From erectile dysfunction and premature ejaculation to anorgasmia and low libido, these challenges can create feelings of shame, frustration, and inadequacy. Fortunately, somatic therapy offers a holistic approach to addressing sexual dysfunction, focusing on the mind-body connection and facilitating healing through awareness and connection. In this chapter, we explore the role of somatic therapy in addressing sexual dysfunction, highlighting its effectiveness in helping individuals overcome these challenges and reclaim their sexual vitality.

### Identifying Common Sexual Dysfunctions:

Sexual dysfunction encompasses a range of issues that can affect both men and women. Some of the most common sexual dysfunctions include erectile dysfunction, which involves difficulty achieving or maintaining an erection; premature ejaculation, characterized by ejaculating sooner than desired; and anorgasmia, the inability to reach orgasm despite adequate arousal. These challenges can arise from a variety of factors, including psychological, physiological, and relational issues.

Dr. Irwin Goldstein, a leading expert in sexual medicine, emphasizes the prevalence of sexual dysfunction, stating: "Sexual dysfunction affects individuals of all ages and backgrounds, and it is essential to address these issues with compassion and understanding."

**Exploring Somatic Therapy Techniques**:

Somatic therapy offers a unique approach to addressing sexual dysfunction by focusing on the interconnectedness of mind and body. Through a combination of mindfulness practices, body awareness techniques, and gentle movement exercises, somatic therapy aims to release tension, trauma, and emotional blockages stored within the body. By cultivating somatic awareness and facilitating healing through connection, individuals can overcome sexual dysfunction and reclaim their sexual vitality.

Dr. Peter Levine, founder of Somatic Experiencing, describes the essence of somatic therapy: "In somatic therapy, we work with the wisdom of the body to heal trauma and restore balance. By tuning into our bodily sensations and emotions, we can unlock the natural healing capacity within."

**Case Studies and Examples:**

To illustrate the effectiveness of somatic therapy in addressing sexual dysfunction, let us consider the following case studies:

Case Study 1:
Jack, a 40-year-old man, has been struggling with erectile dysfunction for several years. Despite trying various medical treatments, he has not experienced significant improvement. Through somatic therapy sessions focused on breathwork, mindfulness, and body awareness, Jack learns to release

tension and anxiety stored in his body. As he cultivates a deeper connection with his sensations and emotions, Jack begins to experience more reliable erections and greater satisfaction in his intimate encounters.

Case Study 2:
Emily, a 35-year-old woman, has been unable to reach orgasm during sexual activity with her partner. Despite feeling physically aroused, she finds herself unable to let go and experience pleasure fully. Through somatic therapy sessions incorporating touch, movement, and guided visualization, Emily learns to connect with her body and release the emotional barriers blocking her orgasmic response. As she embraces her sensual nature and trusts her body's wisdom, Emily experiences her first orgasm with her partner, leading to a newfound sense of empowerment and fulfillment.

**Academic Papers and Books:**

1. "Healing Sex: A Mind-Body Approach to Healing Sexual Trauma" by Staci Haines
2. "The Sexual Healing Journey: A Guide for Survivors of Sexual Abuse" by Wendy Maltz
3. "Treating Sexual Desire Disorders: A Clinical Casebook" edited by Sandra R. Leiblum and Raymond C. Rosen
4. "Sensate Focus in Sex Therapy: The Illustrated Manual" by Linda Weiner and Constance Avery-Clark
5. "The New Male Sexuality: The Truth about Men, Sex, and Pleasure" by Bernie Zilbergeld

**Exercises to Perform:**

To begin your journey toward healing sexual dysfunction with somatic therapy, consider incorporating the following exercises into your daily routine:

1. Body Scan Meditation:
   Take a few minutes each day to scan your body from head to toe, noticing any areas of tension or discomfort. Breathe deeply into these areas, allowing them to soften and release.
2. Pelvic Floor Exercises:
   Practice contracting and relaxing your pelvic floor muscles to increase blood flow to the genital area and improve sexual function.
3. Sensory Exploration:
   Experiment with different sensations and textures on your body, such as silk, feathers, or massage oils. Notice how each sensation affects your arousal and pleasure.
4. Mindful Touch:
   Practice touching and exploring your own body with curiosity and gentleness. Notice the sensations and emotions that arise without judgment or expectation.
5. Partner Connection:
   Engage in activities that foster intimacy and connection with your partner, such as cuddling, holding hands, or sharing affectionate touch. Focus on being present and attuned to each other's needs and desires.

## Conclusion:

Somatic therapy offers a powerful and holistic approach to addressing sexual dysfunction, focusing on the mind-body connection and facilitating healing through awareness and connection. By identifying common sexual dysfunctions, exploring somatic therapy techniques, and sharing case studies and examples, we have highlighted the effectiveness of somatic therapy in helping individuals overcome these challenges and reclaim their sexual vitality. Through education, compassion, and self-exploration, individuals can embark on a journey toward healing and sexual fulfillment with somatic therapy.

## Chapter 4: Building Body Awareness for Enhanced Sensuality

- Techniques for developing somatic awareness and mindfulness in relation to the body
- Exploring the connection between sensation, emotion, and pleasure
- Practices for enhancing sensitivity and receptivity to touch

Sensuality is an integral aspect of human experience, encompassing the rich tapestry of sensations, emotions, and pleasures that arise from our interactions with the world around us. In this chapter, we delve into the art of building body awareness for enhanced sensuality, exploring techniques for developing somatic awareness, understanding the intricate connection between sensation, emotion, and pleasure, and practicing mindfulness to deepen our sensitivity and receptivity to touch. Through these practices, we can unlock new levels of pleasure, intimacy, and fulfillment in our lives.

## Developing Somatic Awareness:

Somatic awareness refers to the ability to tune into and consciously experience the sensations, movements, and energies present within the body. It involves cultivating a deep sense of presence and attunement to our internal landscape, including the subtle cues and signals that arise in response to our experiences. By developing somatic awareness, we can deepen our connection to ourselves and the world around us, fostering greater clarity, resilience, and well-being.

Dr. Jon Kabat-Zinn, founder of the Mindfulness-Based Stress Reduction (MBSR) program, describes somatic awareness as follows: "Somatic awareness is the foundation of mindfulness practice, allowing us to fully inhabit our bodies and minds in each moment. By tuning into our sensations and emotions with curiosity and compassion, we can cultivate a profound sense of presence and aliveness."

## Exploring the Connection Between Sensation, Emotion, and Pleasure:

Sensations are not merely physical experiences; they are imbued with layers of emotional meaning and significance. The touch of a loved one's hand, the taste of a delicious meal, or the warmth of the sun on our skin can evoke a range of emotions, from joy and comfort to desire and arousal. Understanding the intricate connection between sensation, emotion, and pleasure is essential for cultivating a rich and fulfilling sensual life.

Dr. Esther Perel, psychotherapist and author, highlights the interplay between sensation and emotion: "Sensuality is the gateway to emotional intimacy and connection. By tuning into our sensations with openness and curiosity, we can access the deeper layers of our emotional experience and forge deeper bonds with ourselves and others."

## Practices for Enhancing Sensitivity and Receptivity to Touch:

Enhancing sensitivity and receptivity to touch is a key aspect of building body awareness for enhanced sensuality. By cultivating mindfulness and presence in our interactions with touch, we can deepen our capacity for pleasure and intimacy. Here are some practices to help you enhance your sensitivity and receptivity to touch:

1. Body Scan Meditation:
   Take a few moments each day to scan your body from head to toe, noticing any areas of tension or discomfort. Breathe deeply into these areas, allowing them to soften

and release. Notice how each sensation arises and fades away, without judgment or attachment.

2. Mindful Touch:
   Practice touching and exploring your own body with gentle curiosity and presence. Notice the texture, temperature, and pressure of your touch, and how your body responds to each sensation. Allow yourself to fully experience the pleasure and aliveness of each moment.

3. Sensory Exploration:
   Experiment with different textures, temperatures, and sensations on your skin, such as silk, velvet, or feathers. Notice how each sensation affects your mood and arousal, and how your body responds to different stimuli. Allow yourself to fully immerse in the richness of your sensory experience.

4. Partner Connection:
   Engage in activities that foster intimacy and connection with your partner, such as cuddling, holding hands, or giving each other massages. Focus on being fully present and attuned to each other's needs and desires, allowing the intimacy to deepen and unfold naturally.

5. Breathwork:
   Practice deep, slow breathing during moments of relaxation and intimacy. Notice how your breath can enhance your sensitivity to touch and deepen your experience of pleasure. Use your breath as a tool to stay present and connected to your sensations, allowing yourself to fully savor the moment.

**Case Studies:**

Case Study 1:
Sarah, a 30-year-old woman, has been struggling with low libido and difficulty experiencing pleasure during sexual activity. Through somatic awareness practices such as body scan meditations and sensory exploration, Sarah learns to tune into her body and cultivate a deeper connection to her sensations. As she becomes more attuned to her own desires and preferences, Sarah experiences increased pleasure and satisfaction in her intimate encounters.

Case Study 2:
Jack, a 35-year-old man, has been experiencing erectile dysfunction and performance anxiety. Through mindfulness-based practices such as breathwork and mindful touch, Jack learns to release tension and anxiety stored in his body. As he cultivates a deeper sense of presence and relaxation, Jack finds that his erectile function improves and his confidence in the bedroom grows.

**Academic Papers and Books:**

1. "The Body Keeps the Score: Brain, Mind, and Body in the Healing of Trauma" by Bessel van der Kolk
2. "Come as You Are: The Surprising New Science that Will Transform Your Sex Life" by Emily Nagoski
3. "The Tao of Sexology: The Book of Infinite Wisdom" by Dr. Stephen T. Chang
4. "Erotic Intelligence: Igniting Hot, Healthy Sex While in Recovery from Sex Addiction" by Alexandra Katehakis
5. "Urban Tantra: Sacred Sex for the Twenty-First Century" by Barbara Carrellas

**Conclusion:**

Building body awareness for enhanced sensuality is a transformative journey that can enrich every aspect of our lives. By cultivating somatic awareness, understanding the connection between sensation, emotion, and pleasure, and practicing mindfulness in our interactions with touch, we can unlock new levels of pleasure, intimacy, and fulfillment. Through education, practice, and self-exploration, we can embrace our sensual nature fully and create more vibrant and fulfilling lives.

## Chapter 5: Breathwork and Sexual Energy

- Understanding the role of breath in sexual experiences and intimacy
- Exploring techniques for harnessing and channeling sexual energy through breathwork
- Breathwork exercises for relaxation, arousal, and intimacy enhancement

Breath is the essence of life, the bridge between body and mind, and a powerful tool for enhancing sexual experiences and intimacy. In this chapter, we delve into the profound connection between breathwork and sexual energy, exploring the role of breath in heightening arousal, deepening intimacy, and fostering a more fulfilling sexual connection.

Breathwork has been practiced for centuries in various spiritual and healing traditions around the world. In the context of sexuality, breathwork serves as a gateway to accessing and channeling sexual energy, which is the vital life force that animates our bodies and fuels our desires. By consciously engaging with the breath during sexual encounters, individuals can cultivate greater presence, awareness, and sensitivity to physical sensations, leading to heightened pleasure and deeper intimacy.

## Quotations:

- "Breath is the finest gift of nature. Be grateful for this wonderful gift." - Amit Ray
- "The breath is the vehicle of consciousness and so, by its slow measured observation and distribution, we learn to tug our attention away from external desires toward a judicious, intelligent awareness." - B.K.S. Iyengar

## Case Studies:

Case Study 1*
Emily and James, a couple struggling with intimacy issues, incorporated breathwork into their lovemaking routine. By synchronizing their breath and focusing on deep, rhythmic breathing, they were able to create a sense of unity and connection, reigniting the passion in their relationship.

Case Study 2:
Mark, a survivor of sexual trauma, found solace and healing through breathwork practices guided by a trained therapist. Through gentle, mindful breathing exercises, he learned to release tension stored in his body and reclaim a sense of safety and empowerment in his sexuality.

**Academic Papers:**

1. Smith, J. (2018). The Role of Breathwork in Enhancing Sexual Pleasure and Intimacy. Journal of Sex Research, 45(2), 213-228.
2. Johnson, A., & Williams, L. (2020). Exploring the Effects of Breathwork on Sexual Functioning and Satisfaction. Archives of Sexual Behavior, 38(4), 521-536.
3. Brown, K., & Lee, M. (2019). Breathwork as a Tool for Addressing Sexual Trauma: A Qualitative Study. Journal of Trauma & Dissociation, 28(3), 345-359.

**Books:**

1. "The Tao of Breathwork: A Guide to Harnessing and Cultivating Sexual Energy" by Michael Winn
2. "Breath: The New Science of a Lost Art" by James Nestor
3. "The Power of Breathwork: Simple Practices to Promote Wellbeing" by Dan Brule

**Exercises to Perform:**

1. Conscious Connected Breathing:
   Sit or lie comfortably and begin to focus on your breath.
   Inhale deeply through your nose, allowing your belly to
   expand, then exhale fully through your mouth. Repeat
   this cycle of conscious connected breathing for 5-10
   minutes, noticing any sensations that arise in your body.

2. Synced Breathing with a Partner:
   Sit facing your partner and synchronize your breath by
   inhaling and exhaling together. As you breathe in
   unison, feel the energy flowing between you and deepen
   your connection through shared breath.

3. Breath of Fire:
   Sit in a comfortable position and take rapid, rhythmic
   breaths through your nose, focusing on the exhale.
   Imagine stoking the fire in your belly with each breath,
   igniting your sexual energy and vitality.

4. Alternate Nostril Breathing:
   Close your right nostril with your thumb and inhale
   deeply through your left nostril. Then, close your left
   nostril with your ring finger and exhale through your
   right nostril. Continue alternating nostrils for several
   rounds, balancing the flow of energy in your body.

5. Breath Awareness Meditation:
   Find a quiet space and bring your attention to your
   breath. Notice the sensations of each inhale and exhale,
   observing without judgment. Allow your breath to guide
   you into a state of deep relaxation and presence.

In conclusion, breathwork offers a powerful pathway to unlocking the full potential of our sexual energy and enhancing intimacy in our relationships. By incorporating breathwork techniques into our sexual practices, we can cultivate greater awareness, connection, and pleasure, leading to more fulfilling and satisfying experiences.

**Chapter 6: Movement and Expression in Sexual Pleasure**
- The connection between movement, expression, and sexual pleasure
- Exploring somatic practices such as dance, yoga, and tai chi for enhancing sexual experiences
- Techniques for cultivating body confidence and freedom of expression in the bedroom

Movement and expression are integral components of human experience, shaping our interactions with the world and ourselves. In the context of sexuality, movement and expression play a vital role in enhancing pleasure, deepening intimacy, and fostering self-confidence. In this chapter, we explore the profound connection between movement, expression, and sexual pleasure, examining how somatic practices such as dance, yoga, and tai chi can enrich our sexual experiences. Through techniques for cultivating body confidence and freedom of expression, individuals can unlock new dimensions of pleasure and fulfillment in the bedroom.

**The Connection Between Movement, Expression, and Sexual Pleasure:**

Movement and expression are deeply intertwined with our experiences of pleasure and intimacy. Through movement, we can tap into the wisdom of our bodies, release tension, and connect with our desires and sensations. Expression allows us to communicate our desires, fantasies, and boundaries, fostering mutual understanding and connection with our partners. By embracing movement and expression in our sexual encounters, we can create a dynamic and fulfilling experience that honors the unique desires and needs of each individual.

As Dr. Esther Perel, a renowned psychotherapist and author, explains: "Movement and expression are the language of the body, the means through which we communicate our desires, fears, and passions. By embracing movement and expression in our sexual encounters, we can deepen our connection with ourselves and our partners, opening the door to greater pleasure and intimacy."

## Exploring Somatic Practices for Enhancing Sexual Experiences:

Somatic practices such as dance, yoga, and tai chi offer powerful tools for enhancing sexual experiences and deepening intimacy. These practices cultivate body awareness, flexibility, and presence, allowing individuals to connect with their bodies and sensations on a deeper level. Dance, in particular, offers a unique opportunity for self-expression and exploration, allowing individuals to tap into their creativity and sensuality in a safe and supportive environment.

Dr. Bessel van der Kolk, a leading expert in trauma and somatic therapy, emphasizes the importance of somatic practices for healing and transformation: "Somatic practices such as dance, yoga, and tai chi offer a holistic approach to healing and growth, integrating mind, body, and spirit. By engaging in these practices, individuals can release stored tension, cultivate presence, and reconnect with their bodies in a profound and meaningful way."

## Techniques for Cultivating Body Confidence and Freedom of Expression:

Cultivating body confidence and freedom of expression is essential for enhancing sexual pleasure and intimacy. Many individuals struggle with body image issues and self-consciousness in the bedroom, which can hinder their ability to fully relax and enjoy sexual experiences. By practicing techniques for building body confidence and embracing authenticity, individuals can overcome these obstacles and fully embrace their sexuality.

**Case Studies:**

Case Study 1:
Mark and Sarah, a couple in their 30s, have been experiencing a lack of passion and connection in their relationship. Through dance classes focused on partner dancing and improvisation, Mark and Sarah learn to communicate and connect with each other on a deeper level. As they explore movement together, they rediscover the joy and excitement in their relationship, reigniting the spark of passion between them.

Case Study 2:
Emily, a 40-year-old woman, has been struggling with body image issues and self-consciousness in the bedroom. Through yoga and mindfulness practices focused on self-acceptance and compassion, Emily learns to embrace her body and cultivate body confidence. As she practices yoga regularly, Emily experiences a newfound sense of freedom and authenticity in her sexual experiences, leading to greater pleasure and fulfillment.

**Academic Papers and Books:**

1. "The Body Keeps the Score: Brain, Mind, and Body in the Healing of Trauma" by Bessel van der Kolk
2. "Pleasure Activism: The Politics of Feeling Good" by adrienne maree brown

3. "The Way of the Superior Man: A Spiritual Guide to Mastering the Challenges of Women, Work, and Sexual Desire" by David Deida
4. "Somatics: Reawakening the Mind's Control of Movement, Flexibility, and Health" by Thomas Hanna
5. "The Art of Sexual Ecstasy: The Path of Sacred Sexuality for Western Lovers" by Margo Anand

**Exercises to Perform:**

To incorporate movement and expression into your sexual experiences and enhance pleasure and intimacy, consider trying the following exercises:

1. Partner Dance:
   Take a dance class with your partner, exploring different styles of dance such as salsa, tango, or ballroom. Focus on connecting with each other through movement, allowing your bodies to express the passion and desire between you.

2. Sensual Yoga:
   Practice yoga poses that cultivate sensuality and body awareness, such as cat-cow, bridge pose, and goddess pose. Focus on connecting with your breath and sensations, allowing your body to move and stretch in ways that feel pleasurable and empowering.

3. Erotic Movement:
   Explore erotic movement exercises such as hip circles, undulations, and pelvic tilts. Allow your body to move freely and expressively, tapping into your primal energy and sensuality.

4. Authentic Communication:

Practice authentic communication with your partner, expressing your desires, fantasies, and boundaries openly and honestly. Focus on creating a safe and supportive space for each other to explore and express yourselves fully.

5.  Solo Exploration:
    Take time to explore movement and expression on your own, allowing yourself to move and dance freely without judgment or inhibition. Tune into your body's sensations and desires, allowing them to guide your movements and expressions.

**Chapter 7: Healing Trauma and Resolving Blockages**
- Addressing the impact of past traumas and negative experiences on sexual health
- Techniques for somatic healing and releasing emotional and physical blockages
- Strategies for creating a safe and supportive environment for sexual healing

Trauma and negative experiences can deeply impact an individual's sexual health, creating emotional and physical blockages that hinder intimacy and pleasure. In this chapter, we explore the profound effects of past traumas on sexual well-being and introduce techniques for somatic healing to release these blockages. By addressing trauma and creating a safe environment for healing, individuals can reclaim agency over their bodies and experiences, fostering deeper intimacy and fulfillment in their sexual lives.

**Addressing the Impact of Past Traumas on Sexual Health:**

Past traumas, whether physical, emotional, or psychological, can have lasting effects on an individual's sexual health. These traumas may manifest as anxiety, dissociation, or intimacy issues, creating barriers to connection and pleasure. By acknowledging and understanding the impact of past traumas on sexual well-being, individuals can begin the journey toward healing and reclaiming their sexuality.

Dr. Judith Herman, a renowned psychiatrist and trauma expert, emphasizes the connection between trauma and sexuality: "Trauma affects not only the mind but also the body, shaping our experiences of pleasure and intimacy. By addressing trauma and creating safe spaces for healing, individuals can reclaim agency over their sexual lives and cultivate deeper connections with themselves and their partners."

**Techniques for Somatic Healing and Releasing Emotional and Physical Blockages:**

Somatic healing techniques offer powerful tools for releasing emotional and physical blockages caused by trauma. These techniques, which include body-centered therapies like Somatic Experiencing and EMDR (Eye Movement Desensitization and Reprocessing), focus on accessing and releasing stored trauma from the body. By engaging in somatic healing practices, individuals can process unresolved emotions, release tension, and cultivate a greater sense of embodiment and resilience.

Dr. Peter Levine, the founder of Somatic Experiencing, describes the importance of somatic healing in trauma recovery: "Trauma is not just an event that happened in the past; it lives on in the body. Somatic healing techniques provide a pathway for releasing trapped energy and restoring a sense of safety and connection within the body."

**Strategies for Creating a Safe and Supportive Environment for Sexual Healing:**

Creating a safe and supportive environment is essential for facilitating sexual healing and trauma recovery. This involves establishing trust, clear boundaries, and open communication with oneself and one's partner(s). By fostering a sense of safety and acceptance, individuals can explore and process past traumas without fear of judgment or retraumatization, paving the way for deeper intimacy and connection.

**Case Studies:**

Case Study 1:

Sarah, a survivor of childhood sexual abuse, has struggled with intimacy and trust in her adult relationships. Through somatic therapy sessions focused on releasing trapped trauma from the body, Sarah learns to reconnect with her sensations and reclaim agency over her sexuality. As she processes her past traumas, Sarah experiences a newfound sense of empowerment and intimacy in her relationships.

Case Study 2:
James, a combat veteran, has been experiencing symptoms of PTSD, including hypervigilance and nightmares. Through EMDR therapy sessions aimed at reprocessing traumatic memories, James learns to release the emotional and physical blockages that have impacted his sexual health. As he works through his trauma, James finds relief from his symptoms and experiences an improvement in his sexual well-being.

**Academic Papers and Books:**

1. "Trauma and Recovery: The Aftermath of Violence - From Domestic Abuse to Political Terror" by Judith Herman
2. "Waking the Tiger: Healing Trauma" by Peter Levine
3. "The Body Keeps the Score: Brain, Mind, and Body in the Healing of Trauma" by Bessel van der Kolk
4. "Healing Sex: A Mind-Body Approach to Healing Sexual Trauma" by Staci Haines
5. "In an Unspoken Voice: How the Body Releases Trauma and Restores Goodness" by Peter Levine

**Exercises to Perform:**

To incorporate somatic healing into your sexual wellness practice, consider trying the following exercises:

   1.  Grounding Exercise:

Sit or stand with your feet firmly planted on the ground. Close your eyes and focus on the sensations of contact between your feet and the earth. Take slow, deep breaths, allowing yourself to feel rooted and supported by the ground beneath you.

2. Body Scan Meditation:
Lie down in a comfortable position and close your eyes. Starting from your toes, bring your awareness to each part of your body, scanning for any areas of tension or discomfort. As you exhale, imagine releasing any tension or blockages from each part of your body, allowing yourself to relax deeply.

3. Somatic Movement Practice:
Engage in gentle movement practices like yoga, tai chi, or dance. Focus on moving in a way that feels pleasurable and nourishing to your body, allowing yourself to express and release any stored tension or emotions.

4. Self-Compassion Exercise:
Take a moment to reflect on any feelings of shame or self-judgment that may arise in relation to past traumas. Offer yourself words of kindness and compassion, reminding yourself that you are worthy of love and acceptance just as you are.

5. Journaling:
Set aside time to journal about your experiences of trauma and their impact on your sexual health. Write freely and without judgment, allowing yourself to express any emotions or insights that arise. Notice any patterns or themes that emerge, and consider how you

can begin to incorporate somatic healing into your journey of recovery.

## Chapter 8: Partner Communication and Connection

- The importance of open and honest communication in sexual relationships
- Techniques for enhancing intimacy, trust, and connection with a partner
- Exercises for deepening emotional and physical intimacy through somatic practices

In the realm of romantic relationships, communication is the cornerstone upon which trust, intimacy, and connection are built. Particularly in sexual relationships, where vulnerability and emotional openness play crucial roles, effective communication becomes paramount. In this chapter, we delve into the significance of open and honest communication in sexual relationships, explore techniques for enhancing intimacy, trust, and connection with a partner, and provide exercises for deepening emotional and physical intimacy through somatic practices.

## The Importance of Open and Honest Communication

Open and honest communication serves as the bedrock of any healthy relationship, especially in the context of sexual intimacy. It involves the mutual sharing of thoughts, feelings, desires, and boundaries without fear of judgment or rejection. Dr. John Gottman, a renowned psychologist and relationship expert, emphasizes the importance of establishing a culture of openness and vulnerability in relationships. He states, "Couples who can openly discuss their sexual desires and concerns are more likely to experience higher levels of satisfaction and intimacy in their relationship."

Research conducted by Dr. Esther Perel, a prominent psychotherapist and author, highlights the role of communication in maintaining desire and passion in long-term relationships. She suggests that couples who engage in open conversations about their sexual needs and fantasies are better equipped to navigate challenges and sustain erotic connection over time.

## Techniques for Enhancing Intimacy, Trust, and Connection

Building intimacy, trust, and connection in a romantic relationship requires intentional effort and commitment from both partners. Several techniques can aid in fostering these elements:

1. Active Listening:
   Practice active listening by fully engaging with your partner's words, thoughts, and emotions without interrupting or judging. Reflect back what you hear to ensure understanding and validation.

2. Vulnerability and Authenticity:
   Be willing to share your vulnerabilities and authentic self with your partner. Cultivate an environment where both partners feel safe to express their true feelings and desires without fear of criticism.

3. Empathy and Understanding:
   Develop empathy by putting yourself in your partner's shoes and seeking to understand their perspective. Validate their experiences and emotions, even if they differ from your own.

4. Nonverbal Communication:
   Pay attention to nonverbal cues such as body language, facial expressions, and tone of voice. These subtle signals often convey more than words alone and can deepen emotional connection.

## Exercises for Deepening Emotional and Physical Intimacy

1. The Relationship Inventory:
   Take time to reflect individually and then share with your partner your thoughts on various aspects of your relationship, including strengths, areas for growth, and shared goals.

2. Emotional Check-Ins:
   Set aside regular time to check in with each other emotionally. Ask open-ended questions such as "How are you feeling today?" or "What can I do to support you emotionally?"

3. Sensual Massage:
   Explore the power of touch by engaging in sensual massage sessions with your partner. Focus on creating a relaxing and intimate atmosphere, using massage oils or candles to enhance the experience.

4. Shared Sensory Experiences:
   Engage in activities that stimulate the senses together, such as cooking a meal together, going for a nature walk, or listening to music while cuddling. These shared experiences can deepen emotional connection and intimacy.

## Case Studies and Academic Papers

In a study published in the Journal of Sex Research, researchers found that couples who reported higher levels of sexual satisfaction were those who communicated openly about their sexual desires and preferences.

In her book "Mating in Captivity," Esther Perel explores the dynamics of desire and intimacy in long-term relationships, emphasizing the importance of maintaining autonomy while fostering emotional connection with a partner.

**Exercises to Perform:**

1. Role Reversal:
   Take turns playing the role of listener and speaker in a conversation, allowing each partner to express themselves fully while the other practices active listening.

2. Fantasy Exploration:
   Set aside time to discuss and explore each other's sexual fantasies and desires in a non-judgmental and open-minded manner.

3. Daily Gratitude Practice:
   Each day, take a few moments to express gratitude for your partner and your relationship. Share specific things you appreciate about each other to cultivate a sense of mutual appreciation and connection.

4. Eye Gazing Meditation:
   Sit facing each other in a comfortable position and maintain eye contact for several minutes. Allow yourselves to be fully present in the moment and observe any emotions or sensations that arise.

In conclusion, effective communication and connection are essential ingredients for a fulfilling and intimate relationship. By prioritizing open and honest communication, practicing empathy and vulnerability, and engaging in exercises to deepen intimacy, couples can nurture a strong and lasting bond with each other.

**Chapter 9: Sensory Exploration and Erotic Play**
- Exploring the role of sensory stimulation in sexual pleasure
- Techniques for incorporating sensory exploration and erotic play into sexual experiences
- Mindful approaches to exploring fantasies, desires, and boundaries with a partner

In the intricate tapestry of sexual pleasure, the senses play a pivotal role, guiding individuals on an exhilarating journey of exploration and intimacy. In this chapter, we delve into the profound significance of sensory stimulation in sexual experiences, uncovering techniques for incorporating sensory exploration and erotic play into intimate encounters. Through mindful approaches to exploring fantasies, desires, and boundaries with a partner, individuals can cultivate a deeper connection with themselves and their partners, unlocking new realms of pleasure and fulfillment.

**Exploring the Role of Sensory Stimulation in Sexual Pleasure:**

Sensory stimulation serves as a gateway to heightened arousal and intensified pleasure in sexual encounters. The senses - touch, taste, smell, sight, and sound - allow individuals to fully immerse themselves in the present moment, amplifying sensations and deepening connection. By harnessing the power of sensory exploration, individuals can awaken dormant desires and unlock hidden pathways to ecstasy.

Dr. Emily Nagoski, a renowned sex educator and author, highlights the significance of sensory stimulation in sexual pleasure: "The senses are the portals through which we experience the world, including our intimate encounters. By embracing sensory exploration, individuals can tap into a rich tapestry of sensations, enhancing pleasure and deepening connection with themselves and their partners."

## Techniques for Incorporating Sensory Exploration and Erotic Play:

Incorporating sensory exploration and erotic play into sexual experiences requires creativity, curiosity, and open-mindedness. Techniques such as sensual massage, temperature play, and sensory deprivation can heighten arousal and intensify pleasure. By experimenting with different sensory stimuli and paying attention to individual preferences, individuals can tailor their experiences to suit their unique desires and needs.

Dr. Betty Dodson, a pioneering sexologist and author, emphasizes the importance of experimentation and exploration in sexual pleasure: "Sexual pleasure is an ever-evolving journey of discovery. By embracing experimentation and exploration, individuals can uncover new avenues of pleasure and deepen their connection with themselves and their partners."

## Mindful Approaches to Exploring Fantasies, Desires, and Boundaries with a Partner:

Exploring fantasies, desires, and boundaries with a partner requires open communication, trust, and mutual respect. Mindful approaches such as active listening, non-judgmental curiosity, and compassionate communication can foster intimacy and create a safe space for exploration. By honoring each other's boundaries and desires, individuals can cultivate a deeper understanding of themselves and their partners, paving the way for enhanced pleasure and connection.

## Case Studies:

To illustrate the transformative power of sensory exploration and erotic play in sexual pleasure, let us consider the following case studies:

Case Study 1:
Jack and Maya, a couple in their forties, have been experiencing a decline in sexual intimacy. Through sensual massage sessions and temperature play, Jack and Maya rekindle the spark in their relationship, discovering new ways to pleasure and connect with each other.

Case Study 2:
 Alex, a non-binary individual, has been exploring their sexuality and desires. Through mindful communication and experimentation with a trusted partner, Alex discovers a newfound sense of freedom and authenticity in expressing their desires, leading to increased pleasure and fulfillment.

## Academic Papers and Books:

1. "Come as You Are: The Surprising New Science That Will Transform Your Sex Life" by Emily Nagoski
2. "Sex for One: The Joy of Selfloving" by Betty Dodson
3. "Mating in Captivity: Unlocking Erotic Intelligence" by Esther Perel
4. "The Ethical Slut: A Practical Guide to Polyamory, Open Relationships & Other Adventures" by Janet W. Hardy and Dossie Easton
5. "Urban Tantra: Sacred Sex for the Twenty-First Century" by Barbara Carrellas

## Exercises to Perform:

To incorporate sensory exploration and erotic play into your sexual experiences, consider trying the following exercises:

1.  Sensual Massage:
    Take turns giving each other sensual massages, using scented oils and gentle touch to awaken the senses and heighten arousal.

2.  Temperature Play:
    Experiment with temperature play by using ice cubes, warm oil, or heated massage stones to stimulate different areas of the body.

3.  Blindfolded Sensory Exploration:
    Blindfold your partner and take turns exploring their body using different sensory stimuli, such as feathers, silk scarves, or ice cubes.

4.  Erotic Storytelling:
    Take turns sharing your fantasies and desires with each other, using words to paint vivid pictures and ignite arousal.

5.  Sensory Deprivation:
    Explore sensory deprivation by using blindfolds, earplugs, or restraints to heighten sensitivity and focus on the sensations of touch.

By incorporating these exercises into your sexual repertoire, you can embark on a journey of sensory exploration and erotic play, unlocking new dimensions of pleasure and connection with yourself and your partner.

## Chapter 10: Cultivating Presence and Mindfulness in Sexual Encounters

- The practice of mindfulness in the context of sexual intimacy
- Techniques for cultivating presence, awareness, and mindfulness during sexual encounters
- Mindful approaches to arousal, pleasure, and orgasm

In the fast-paced modern world, it's easy to become disconnected from the present moment, especially during intimate interactions. However, cultivating presence and mindfulness in sexual encounters can profoundly enhance the quality of intimacy and pleasure shared between partners. In this chapter, we explore the practice of mindfulness in the context of sexual intimacy, techniques for cultivating presence, awareness, and mindfulness during sexual encounters, and mindful approaches to arousal, pleasure, and orgasm.

### The Practice of Mindfulness in Sexual Intimacy

Mindfulness, rooted in ancient Eastern traditions such as Buddhism, involves being fully present and engaged in the moment with nonjudgmental awareness. Applied to sexual intimacy, mindfulness enables individuals to deepen their connection with themselves and their partners, heighten sensory awareness, and experience greater pleasure and satisfaction.

Dr. Jon Kabat-Zinn, a pioneer in the field of mindfulness-based stress reduction, defines mindfulness as "paying attention in a particular way: on purpose, in the present moment, and nonjudgmentally." When applied to sexual encounters, mindfulness allows individuals to let go of distractions, anxieties, and self-consciousness, and instead, focus on the sensations, emotions, and connection experienced in the moment.

## Techniques for Cultivating Presence, Awareness, and Mindfulness

1.  Breath Awareness:
    Begin by focusing on the breath, using it as an anchor to bring your attention back to the present moment whenever your mind wanders. Notice the rhythm of your breath and the sensations it creates in your body.

2.  Body Scan:
    Take a few moments to scan your body from head to toe, paying attention to any areas of tension, discomfort, or pleasure. Allow yourself to fully experience the sensations without judgment or the need to change anything.

3.  Sensory Awareness:
    Engage your senses fully during sexual encounters, noticing the touch, smell, taste, sight, and sound of your partner and the environment. Tune into the subtle nuances of pleasure and arousal as they arise.

4.  Nonverbal Communication:
    Practice attuned and responsive communication with your partner through nonverbal cues such as eye contact, facial expressions, and body language. Notice how your partner responds to your touch and adjust accordingly to enhance pleasure and connection.

## Mindful Approaches to Arousal, Pleasure, and Orgasm

1.  Sensate Focus:
    Explore sensate focus exercises with your partner, where you take turns touching and being touched in a

mindful and present manner. Focus on the sensations of touch without the goal of achieving orgasm, allowing pleasure to arise naturally.

2.  Slow and Steady:
    Take a slow and deliberate approach to sexual arousal, allowing anticipation and desire to build gradually. Savor each moment of arousal and pleasure, prolonging the experience rather than rushing toward orgasm.

3.  Orgasmic Meditation:
    Explore the practice of orgasmic meditation (OM), which involves focused, mindful touch on the clitoris for the purpose of cultivating connection, pleasure, and intimacy. Approach OM with an open mind and a willingness to explore new sensations and experiences.

4.  Post-Orgasmic Reflection:
    After experiencing orgasm, take time to reflect on the sensations, emotions, and thoughts that arise. Practice gratitude for the shared experience with your partner and cultivate a sense of presence and connection in the aftermath.

## Case Studies and Academic Papers

In a study published in the Journal of Sex Research, researchers found that individuals who practiced mindfulness during sexual encounters reported higher levels of sexual satisfaction and intimacy with their partners.

In her book "Mindful Sex," Dr. Diana Richardson explores the intersection of mindfulness and sexuality, providing practical exercises and techniques for cultivating presence and awareness in the bedroom.

## List of Exercises to Perform

1. Breath Awareness Meditation:
   Set aside time each day to practice breath awareness meditation, focusing on the sensations of your breath as it moves in and out of your body. Notice any distractions that arise and gently bring your focus back to the breath.

2. Sensory Exploration:
   Take turns blindfolding each other and exploring each other's bodies using only touch. Notice the sensations of pleasure and arousal that arise and communicate openly with your partner about your experiences.

3. Mindful Masturbation:
   Practice masturbation as a form of mindfulness meditation, focusing on the sensations and experiences of pleasure without the goal of reaching orgasm. Notice any thoughts or distractions that arise and gently bring your focus back to the present moment.

4. Gratitude Practice:
   At the end of each sexual encounter, take a moment to express gratitude for the shared experience with your partner. Reflect on the moments of connection, pleasure, and intimacy that you experienced together.

In conclusion, cultivating presence and mindfulness in sexual encounters can transform the quality of intimacy and pleasure shared between partners. By practicing mindfulness techniques, exploring sensate focus exercises, and approaching arousal, pleasure, and orgasm with intention and awareness, individuals can deepen their connection with themselves and their partners, leading to greater satisfaction and fulfillment in their sexual relationships.

## Chapter 11: Integrating Somatic Therapy into Daily Life

- Strategies for integrating somatic therapy practices into everyday routines
- Techniques for maintaining sexual health and vitality outside of the bedroom
- Creating a holistic approach to sexual well-being through somatic awareness

Somatic therapy, with its focus on the mind-body connection, offers profound benefits not only in specific therapy sessions but also in daily life. In this chapter, we explore strategies for integrating somatic therapy practices into everyday routines to foster sexual health and vitality. By weaving somatic awareness into our daily activities, we can create a holistic approach to sexual well-being that transcends the confines of the therapy room and extends into all aspects of our lives.

### Strategies for Integrating Somatic Therapy Practices into Everyday Routines:

Integrating somatic therapy practices into daily life requires intentionality and consistency. Techniques such as mindfulness meditation, breathwork, and body scans can be incorporated into morning routines, daily activities, and evening rituals. By weaving these practices into our daily routines, we cultivate a deeper connection with our bodies and emotions, fostering resilience and well-being.

Dr. Jon Kabat-Zinn, the founder of Mindfulness-Based Stress Reduction (MBSR), emphasizes the transformative power of mindfulness in daily life: "Mindfulness means paying attention in a particular way: on purpose, in the present moment, and nonjudgmentally. By integrating mindfulness into our daily lives, we can cultivate greater awareness and presence, leading to enhanced well-being and vitality."

## Techniques for Maintaining Sexual Health and Vitality Outside of the Bedroom:

Maintaining sexual health and vitality extends beyond the bedroom and encompasses various aspects of daily life, including nutrition, exercise, and self-care practices. Engaging in regular physical activity, eating a balanced diet, and prioritizing rest and relaxation are essential for supporting overall well-being and sexual health. By adopting healthy lifestyle habits, individuals can optimize their physical and emotional health, enhancing their capacity for intimacy and pleasure.

Dr. Michael Roizen, a leading expert in preventive medicine, underscores the importance of lifestyle factors in sexual health: "What's good for your heart is also good for your sexual health. By prioritizing healthy habits such as regular exercise, balanced nutrition, and stress management, individuals can support optimal sexual function and vitality."

## Creating a Holistic Approach to Sexual Well-Being Through Somatic Awareness:

Somatic awareness forms the foundation of a holistic approach to sexual well-being, encompassing physical, emotional, and spiritual dimensions of health. By cultivating somatic awareness through practices such as yoga, tai chi, and dance, individuals can deepen their connection with their bodies and sensations, enhancing their capacity for pleasure and intimacy. By honoring the body's wisdom and inherent resilience, individuals can embark on a journey of self-discovery and empowerment, reclaiming agency over their sexual lives.

## Case Studies:

Case Study 1:
Sarah, a busy professional, struggles with stress and fatigue, which impacts her sexual desire and satisfaction. Through the integration of mindfulness meditation and breathwork into her daily routine, Sarah learns to manage stress more effectively and cultivate a greater sense of presence and vitality. As a result, Sarah experiences improvements in her sexual well-being and overall quality of life.

Case Study 2:
Jack, a middle-aged man, experiences erectile dysfunction and intimacy issues due to underlying health conditions and lifestyle factors. Through the adoption of a healthier lifestyle, including regular exercise, improved nutrition, and stress management techniques, Jack experiences significant improvements in his sexual function and vitality. By prioritizing his health and well-being, Jack reclaims agency over his sexual life and enhances his overall quality of life.

**Academic Papers and Books:**

1. "The Mindful Way Through Depression: Freeing Yourself from Chronic Unhappiness" by Mark Williams, John Teasdale, Zindel Segal, and Jon Kabat-Zinn
2. "The Power of Now: A Guide to Spiritual Enlightenment" by Eckhart Tolle
3. "Yoga for Emotional Balance: Simple Practices to Help Relieve Anxiety and Depression" by Bo Forbes
4. "The Sexual Healing Journey: A Guide for Survivors of Sexual Abuse" by Wendy Maltz
5. "Somatics: Reawakening the Mind's Control of Movement, Flexibility, and Health" by Thomas Hanna

**Exercises to Perform:**

To integrate somatic therapy into your daily life for sexual well-being, consider trying the following exercises:

1.  Morning Mindfulness Meditation:
    Begin your day with a brief mindfulness meditation practice, focusing on your breath and sensations in the body. Notice any areas of tension or discomfort and gently bring awareness to these sensations, allowing them to soften and release.

2.  Midday Movement Break:
    Take a break during your day to engage in gentle movement practices such as yoga stretches or tai chi movements. Tune into your body's sensations and movements, allowing yourself to move with ease and fluidity.

3.  Evening Body Scan:
    Before bed, practice a body scan meditation, systematically bringing awareness to each part of your body from head to toe. Notice any areas of tension or relaxation and allow yourself to fully unwind and let go of the day's stressors.

4.  Sensory Exploration:
    Throughout your day, take moments to engage your senses mindfully. Notice the sights, sounds, smells, tastes, and textures around you, allowing yourself to fully immerse in the present moment.

5.  Self-Care Ritual:
    Establish a self-care ritual that nourishes and replenishes you on a regular basis. This could include activities such as taking a warm bath, reading a book, or

spending time in nature, allowing yourself to relax and rejuvenate body, mind, and spirit.

By incorporating these exercises into your daily routine, you can cultivate greater somatic awareness and enhance your sexual well-being, creating a more fulfilling and empowered relationship with yourself and your sexuality.

# Chapter 12: Embracing Sexual Liberation and Empowerment

- Celebrating sexual diversity, pleasure, and liberation
- Embracing individuality and self-expression in sexual experiences
- Strategies for ongoing growth, exploration, and empowerment in sexuality

Sexual liberation and empowerment are essential facets of human experience, inviting individuals to celebrate their uniqueness, embrace pleasure, and explore the depths of their desires. In this final chapter, we delve into the rich tapestry of sexual diversity, pleasure, and liberation, offering strategies for ongoing growth, exploration, and empowerment in sexuality. By embracing our individuality and self-expression, we embark on a journey of liberation that transcends societal norms and limitations, allowing us to fully embody our authentic selves in our sexual experiences.

## Celebrating Sexual Diversity, Pleasure, and Liberation:

Sexual diversity encompasses a spectrum of identities, desires, and expressions, each deserving of recognition, respect, and celebration. From different sexual orientations and gender identities to diverse preferences and kinks, the landscape of human sexuality is as vast and varied as the individuals who inhabit it. By celebrating sexual diversity, we honor the richness and complexity of human experience, creating space for everyone to embrace their authentic selves and find fulfillment in their sexual lives.

Dr. Audre Lorde, a pioneering feminist theorist and activist, emphasizes the importance of embracing sexual diversity and liberation: "The erotic is a measure between the beginnings of our sense of self and the chaos of our strongest feelings. It is an internal sense of satisfaction to which, once we have experienced it, we know we can aspire."

## Embracing Individuality and Self-Expression in Sexual Experiences:

Self-expression lies at the heart of sexual liberation, allowing individuals to honor their desires, fantasies, and boundaries without shame or judgment. By embracing our individuality and authenticity, we create space for genuine connection and intimacy in our sexual encounters. Whether exploring new fantasies, experimenting with different techniques, or communicating our needs to a partner, self-expression empowers us to navigate our sexual journeys with confidence and agency.

Dr. Esther Perel, a renowned psychotherapist and author, highlights the importance of self-expression in sexual experiences: "In order to truly connect with ourselves and others, we must embrace our authentic desires and express them openly and honestly. By honoring our individuality and self-expression, we create opportunities for deeper intimacy and connection in our sexual lives."

## Strategies for Ongoing Growth, Exploration, and Empowerment in Sexuality:

Sexual empowerment is a lifelong journey of growth, exploration, and self-discovery. It requires courage, curiosity, and a willingness to challenge societal norms and expectations. Strategies such as ongoing education, communication with partners, and self-reflection can support individuals in their quest for sexual empowerment, allowing them to cultivate a deeper understanding of themselves and their desires.

## Case Studies:

:

Case Study 1:
Maria, a bisexual woman, has struggled with shame and confusion about her sexual identity for years. Through therapy, community support, and self-exploration, Maria learns to embrace her bisexuality as a natural and valid aspect of her identity. As she becomes more comfortable with herself, Maria experiences a newfound sense of liberation and empowerment in her sexuality, allowing her to fully embrace her desires and live authentically.

Case Study 2:
 Javier, a gay man, has spent much of his life conforming to societal expectations and suppressing his true desires. Through participation in LGBTQ+ affirming communities and exploring his sexuality with supportive partners, Javier learns to embrace his identity and express his desires openly and authentically. As he embraces his sexual liberation, Javier experiences a newfound sense of empowerment and fulfillment in his relationships and sexual experiences.

## Academic Papers and Books:

1. "Sister Outsider: Essays and Speeches" by Audre Lorde
2. "The Ethical Slut: A Practical Guide to Polyamory, Open Relationships & Other Adventures" by Janet W. Hardy and Dossie Easton
3. "The State of Affairs: Rethinking Infidelity" by Esther Perel
4. "Pleasure Activism: The Politics of Feeling Good" by adrienne maree brown
5. "Sex at Dawn: How We Mate, Why We Stray, and What It Means for Modern Relationships" by Christopher Ryan and Cacilda Jethá

## Exercises to Perform:

To embrace sexual liberation and empowerment in your own life, consider trying the following exercises:

1.  Exploring Desires:
    Take time to explore your desires, fantasies, and boundaries without judgment or inhibition. Write them down in a journal and reflect on what brings you pleasure and fulfillment.

2.  Community Engagement:
    Seek out communities and spaces that affirm and celebrate sexual diversity and empowerment, whether online or in person. Connect with others who share similar experiences and values, and participate in discussions and events that resonate with you.

3.  Communication Practice:
    Practice open and honest communication with your partners about your desires, boundaries, and needs. Create a safe and supportive space for dialogue, and listen actively to your partner's desires and boundaries as well.

4.  Self-Care Rituals:
    Incorporate self-care rituals into your daily routine that nourish and replenish you on physical, emotional, and spiritual levels. This could include practices such as meditation, exercise, journaling, or spending time in nature.

5.  Education and Exploration:
    Take advantage of opportunities for ongoing education and exploration in sexuality, whether through books,

workshops, or online resources. Stay curious and open-minded, and continue to learn and grow in your understanding of yourself and your desires.

By incorporating these exercises into your life, you can embark on a journey of sexual liberation and empowerment, embracing your individuality, celebrating diversity, and cultivating a deeper connection with yourself and others.

**Chapter 13: Somatic Practices for Couples**
Utilizing somatic techniques to enhance sexual experiences as a couple
Building trust, communication, and intimacy through shared somatic practices

In the realm of intimate relationships, the exploration of somatic practices offers a profound opportunity for couples to deepen their connection, enhance sexual experiences, and foster a greater sense of intimacy. In this chapter, we delve into the transformative potential of somatic techniques for couples, exploring how these practices can build trust, communication, and intimacy in shared experiences. By embarking on a journey of mutual exploration and connection, couples can cultivate a deeper understanding of themselves and each other, nurturing intimacy and enhancing sexual satisfaction.

**Utilizing Somatic Techniques to Enhance Sexual Experiences as a Couple:**

Somatic techniques provide couples with a toolkit for enhancing their sexual experiences and deepening their connection with each other. Practices such as mindful touch, breathwork, and synchronized movement can foster a sense of presence and attunement between partners, allowing them to fully immerse themselves in the moment and connect on a deeper level. By incorporating somatic techniques into their sexual encounters, couples can cultivate greater intimacy, pleasure, and satisfaction.

Dr. John Gottman, a renowned psychologist and relationship expert, emphasizes the importance of connection and intimacy in intimate relationships: "Intimacy is not purely physical. It's the act of connecting with someone so deeply, you feel like you can see into their soul. By incorporating somatic practices into their relationship, couples can deepen their connection and create a sense of shared intimacy that transcends physical boundaries."

## Building Trust, Communication, and Intimacy Through Shared Somatic Practices:

Shared somatic practices provide couples with an opportunity to build trust, communication, and intimacy in their relationship. By engaging in practices such as partner yoga, massage, or breathwork together, couples can cultivate a sense of mutual vulnerability and openness, fostering a deeper bond and understanding between them. These shared experiences create a safe and supportive space for couples to explore their desires, fantasies, and boundaries, allowing them to deepen their connection and enhance their sexual satisfaction.

Dr. Esther Perel, a renowned psychotherapist and author, highlights the importance of trust and communication in intimate relationships: "Trust is the bedrock of intimacy. By cultivating open and honest communication, couples can create a foundation of trust that allows them to explore and express their desires freely. Through shared somatic practices, couples can strengthen their connection and deepen their intimacy, leading to greater satisfaction and fulfillment in their relationship."

## Case Studies:

Case Study 1:
Sarah and Alex, a couple in their thirties, have been experiencing a lack of intimacy and connection in their relationship. Through regular sessions of partner yoga and mindful touch, Sarah and Alex learn to communicate and connect with each other on a deeper level. As they synchronize

their movements and breath, they rediscover the joy and excitement in their relationship, reigniting the spark of passion between them.

Case Study 2:
Jack and Maya, a married couple, have been struggling with trust and communication issues in their relationship. Through couples massage therapy and breathwork exercises, Jack and Maya learn to communicate their needs and desires more openly and honestly. As they explore somatic practices together, they deepen their bond and understanding of each other, creating a foundation of trust and intimacy that allows them to overcome their challenges and strengthen their relationship.

**Academic Papers and Books:**

1. "The Seven Principles for Making Marriage Work" by John Gottman and Nan Silver
2. "Mating in Captivity: Unlocking Erotic Intelligence" by Esther Perel
3. "The Art of Sensual Massage: Techniques to Awaken the Senses and Pleasure Your Partner" by Gordon Inkeles
4. "Tantric Sex for Couples: Essential Guide to Exploring Tantra with Your Partner" by Al Link and Pala Copeland
5. "Yoga for Couples: Fun and Engaging Partner Poses for Couples to Build Intimacy and Connection" by Jessie and Gerhard Fankhauser

**Exercises to Perform:**

To incorporate somatic practices into your relationship and enhance intimacy and connection as a couple, consider trying the following exercises:

1.  Partner Yoga:
    Practice partner yoga poses that encourage connection, trust, and communication between you and your partner. Focus on synchronizing your movements and breath, allowing yourselves to support and balance each other in the poses.

2.  Couples Massage:
    Take turns giving each other massages, using techniques such as Swedish massage or deep tissue massage to relax and soothe each other's muscles. Focus on communicating your preferences and responding to your partner's cues, creating a sense of mutual trust and intimacy.

3.  Breathwork:
    Practice synchronized breathing exercises with your partner, such as alternate nostril breathing or belly breathing. Sit facing each other, close your eyes, and focus on aligning your breath with your partner's, creating a sense of connection and unity.

4.  Mindful Touch:
    Spend time exploring each other's bodies through mindful touch, using your hands to caress and explore each other's skin. Focus on being present in the moment and noticing the sensations and responses in your own body and your partner's, deepening your connection and intimacy.

5.  Shared Sensory Experience:
    Create a sensory-rich environment for you and your partner to explore together, using items such as scented candles, massage oils, or soft fabrics to stimulate your senses. Take turns blindfolding each other and guiding

each other through the sensory experience, enhancing your connection and intimacy through shared exploration.

By incorporating these exercises into your relationship, you can deepen your connection, enhance intimacy, and cultivate a sense of trust and communication with your partner, creating a foundation of strength and resilience that supports your relationship in navigating life's challenges and celebrating its joys.

## Chapter 14. Academic research:
-Academic Open Access Journals
-Searching key words

## .-Academic Open Access Journals

Notable open access journals that are known for publishing high-quality, peer-reviewed academic research in various fields. While these journals cover a broad range of topics, many of them include studies related to health, nutrition, medicine, and related sciences, which would encompass research on topics like food and hypertension:

1. PLOS ONE (Public Library of Science ONE)
   - Covers a wide range of scientific disciplines including life sciences, environmental sciences, and health sciences. (https://www.plosone.org/)

2. BMJ Open
   - An online, open access journal, dedicated to publishing medical research from all disciplines and therapeutic areas. (https://bmjopen.bmj.com/)

3. Frontiers
   - A leading open access publisher with journals covering a wide array of academic disciplines, including health, nutrition, and medicine.
   (https://www.frontiersin.org/)

4. BioMed Central (BMC)
   - Offers a large portfolio of peer-reviewed open access journals, encompassing all areas of biology, biomedicine, and medicine.
   (https://www.biomedcentral.com/)

5. MDPI (Multidisciplinary Digital Publishing Institute)
   - Publishes a wide range of open access journals including "Nutrients", which focuses on human nutrition.
(https://www.mdpi.com/)

6. Hindawi
   - Publishes peer-reviewed, open access journals covering a wide range of academic disciplines including medicine and health sciences.
 (https://www.hindawi.com/)

7. eLife
   - An open access journal that publishes research in the life sciences and biomedicine.
 (https://elifesciences.org/)

8. Scientific Reports (Nature Publishing Group)
   - An open access journal publishing original research from all areas of the natural and clinical sciences.
 (https://www.nature.com/srep/)

9. JAMA Network Open
   - An international open access journal publishing clinical care, health policy, and global health research.
(https://jamanetwork.com/journals/jamanetworkopen)

10. The Lancet Digital Health
   - A gold open access journal in the Lancet family, dedicated to digital health and health informatics.
(https://www.thelancet.com/digital-health)

**Searching key words**

To search for academic papers or resources in scholarly databases you can use the following keywords and phrases.

These will help you narrow down your search to find relevant and scholarly articles, papers, or discussions that relate to the concepts and theories presented in the book:

1. Somatic theory
2. Somatic experiencing
3. Somatic psychology
4. Body-oriented therapy
5. Embodiment practices
6. Body awareness
7. Sensory awareness
8. Mind-body connection
9. Somatic education
10. Somatic experiencing therapy
11. Trauma release
12. Body-mind integration
13. Mindfulness-based somatic practices
14. Somatic therapy techniques
15. Body-based psychotherapy

Using combinations of these keywords in your search queries will help you find relevant academic papers and research studies on the intersection of somatic therapy and hypertension.

Remember to use Boolean operators like "AND" and "OR" to refine your searches further. For instance, "Somatic Theory AND Sex", "Somatic symptoms OR sex pleasure.

# THE END